How to make herbal teas and heal your body naturally

Jessica Ross

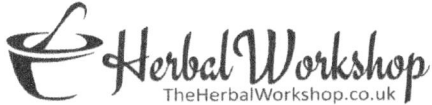

Copyright © 2013 Jessica Ross

All rights reserved.

ISBN-13: 978-1500201135
ISBN-10: 1500201138

Disclaimer

These herbal uses and properties are only given for reference purposes. I am not responsible for any actions or outcome of use of these remedies, taken by persons using these references.

Please be aware that like food a person may have a personal reaction to a herb that is not necessarily a toxic substance. If not sure what the uses and dosages of herbs to be used are please consult a medical or holistic practitioner.

Information provided is not designed to diagnose, prescribe, or treat any illness or injury and is provided for informational purposes only.

Always consult a medical doctor, or other alternative medical practitioner when suffering from any disease, illness, or injury, or before attempting a traditional or folk remedy.

Keep all products away from children. As with any natural product, they can be toxic if misused.

TABLE OF CONTENTS

Welcome _____ 8

Introduction _____ 10

What are the most common herbs? _____ 14

Why use herbal teas? _____ 18

How to make herbal tea _____ 22

Herbal Tea Recipes _____ 24

   All Over Immunity _____ 25

   Allergy Shield _____ 26

   Aphrodite's Secret _____ 27

   Blood Booster _____ 28

   Blooming Healthy _____ 29

   Blues Tea _____ 30

   Calm Waters _____ 31

   Colds and Flu Tea _____ 32

   Dry, raspy cough _____ 33

   Detoxification Tea _____ 34

   Epilepsy Combination _____ 35

Fever Reducer Tea _____ 36

Fluid Retention Tea _____ 37

Happy Man Tea Blend _____ 38

Happy Tummy Tea _____ 39

Heartburn Tea_____ 40

Less Stress Tea _____ 41

Memory Zest Blend _____ 42

Nausea Tea _____ 43

Nervous Stomach Tea_____ 44

Quiet Time Tea _____ 45

Sleep Tea Recipe_____ 46

Sore throat _____ 47

Super Relaxer Tea _____ 48

Tea for Health _____ 49

Tea for menstrual problems, fertility and childbirth. 50

Upset Stomach Tea_____ 51

Winter Tea _____ 52

Very Odd Cure for Bad Breath _____ 53

Bonus herbal smoothie recipes _____ 55

   Berry Basil Green _____ 56

   Raspberry Rosemary_____ 57

   Strawberry Mint Green _____ 58

   Hot and Spicy Green _____ 59

Get Your 100% Free Recipes & Formulations _____ 60

Welcome

Are you curious about herbal tea but worried that you don't know enough to enjoy the numerous health benefits they imbue, instead of just the delicious taste of herbal teas?

Maybe you'd like to start using herbal teas as all natural remedies for your well being, but you're not quite ready to enter the enormous and often confusing world of homeopathy?

Drinking herbal tea is a good way to start treating your ailments naturally and effectively, using simple and cheap herbs, which you probably have some of in your kitchen already. Most, if not all, herbs, spices, berries and roots in this book are easy to get hold of either online or from your grocery store. I've even ensured that the recipes are easy to create no matter if you live in Canada, America or England.

It's not about the simplicity or the taste though; I believe that the secret in creating great herbal teas lies in the ingredients you choose to work with. That's why this book gives you the option for using organic or traditionally grown ingredients in all of our formulations - the results are as important as flavor after all.

Herbal teas mean a lot to me, and indeed The Herbal Workshop too. I've tried to include the widest range of delicious fruit & herbal recipes to start you on your road to discovering the bountiful and amazing benefits of herbal tea. I've not stopped there however, I know that once you try the recipes in this book that you will be hooked, so I'm constantly working on new recipes for you to enjoy, which you can get for free each and every week.

To get your free recipes and much, much more, simply head on over to:

http://ross.theherbalworkshop.co.uk

And send us your email and first name and I will ensure that you get fantastic value for money with ongoing, free recipes and formulations.

Are you ready to enter the exciting world of making your own herbal teas at home with leaves, berries, herbs or flowers of your choice and start drinking these great tasting herbal teas today?

Yours Truly,

Jessica Ross

Introduction

As with any new book, it's often most difficult to find how to start it, and this one is no exception. Herbal teas are such a huge subject that in order to give you the most from a shorter book, that you can digest easily and get making your teas in the same day, I'll skip the 'why' and 'how' the herbs work. Instead I'll focus on getting you the biggest benefit from your time, finding and making the recipe that works for you!

So I'll begin this particular book with this in mind – the herbal tea that you are about to learn to make, with so much acclaim for its health benefits, isn't a tea at all! Well at least not in the strictest sense of the word. The traditional breakfast cup of tea and indeed almost all real 'tea' is made from the leaves of the Camellia sinensis plant, also known as the tea bush. Our herbal tea on the other hand, is more typically an infusion of herbs or flowers so if we were to be pedantic about it, the correct name for it is tisane.

Tisanes are made from the mixtures you will find in this book, typically dried leaves, seeds, grasses, nuts, barks, fruits, flowers, or almost any other botanical element that provide the benefits of your typical herbal teas.

However herbal tea looks just like 'normal' tea and is brewed in the exact same way so I prefer calling it herbal tea.

Unlike other forms of tea though, herbal teas contain no caffeine. I'll state that again, no caffeine. This is great for those on a caffeine free diet for whatever reason. I personally think that they also taste great and are easy to drink. Your tea could consist of just one main herbal ingredient or most likely it will be a blend of specific herbal ingredients, designed for their symbiotic effects and to bring about a specific reaction, such as relaxation, rejuvenation or relief from a specific condition.

For many years now, over a decade to be exact, herbal teas have been 'all the rage' for the vast array of medicinal qualities they are purported to possess. It's commonly claimed they can help with everything from the common cold to fighting Cancer and HIV. While they do posses some astounding properties, much of what you read is hyped up media drivel, designed to sell you a particular product or course.

However, the cold hard fact is that herbal tea, when used correctly, will help in many ailments and illnesses, but sadly cannot cure Cancer or HIV; the plant that holds those secrets hasn't been found – yet!

That doesn't dilute the fact that people have been drinking herbal tea for many Centuries, despite whether or not they knew or understand its benefits for their health. Many types of herbal teas have been widely used as ancient health remedies in Chinese medicine, Ancient Egyptian medicine and as folk remedies on virtually all continents of the World.

Though despite herbal tea obviously helps illness and we have millions of people drinking it every day, science has yet to catch up with any proof that all of the benefits of consuming herbal tea are real. That isn't to say there is no proof; there is more than enough anecdotal evidence from the millions of herbal tea drinkers worldwide over the last Millennia that has been collected to encourage everyone to enjoy a cup when they require it.

The real problem comes from the endless kinds of herbal tea remedies available. Most have a myriad of valuable uses according to traditional folk medicine and of course ancient uses. Chamomile tea has enjoyed more than its fair share of the limelight, and has been one of the best and most studied herbal teas in modern medicine. Because of this, its use as a sleep remedy is well known to all. It can be taken internally or used in a hot bath to help relax you into a restful state and prepare your body for sleep.

Tea has been heralded as the most popular drink in the world, and it's for good reason: your typical herbal teas offer a vast range of health benefits. These concentrated, nutrient rich packages are available in the form of herbal teabags, loose-leaf tea and dried herbs.

Although herbal teabags are available quite easily in supermarkets, it's always a lot more fun to make your own antioxidant-rich beverages at home with leaves, berries, herbs or flowers of your choice.

If using teabags though and I hope you don't, when choosing a herbal tea remedy, ensure you pick the right one. Although fruit flavored teas - such as rosehip, apple and orange - are delicious, they are purely developed for their taste more than anything else.

Herbal teas on the other hand, such as thyme, peppermint and ginger have greater therapeutic virtues as discussed later in the book.

What are the most common herbs?

There are hundreds, if not thousands of different herbs that can be found in herbal teas, each with its own unique use. Some of the really common ones include:

Allspice – helps to soothe the common cold and relieves upset stomachs

Anise seed – aids digestion and freshens the breath. It can also soothe a cough and improve bronchitis.

Bergamot – fights depression and aids digestion

Chamomile – is renowned for its calming properties and is also said to be anti-inflammatory and anti-spasmodic

Chrysanthemum – is sweet-tasting and is able to reduce body heat resulting from fever. It also helps protect against liver damage and neutralizes toxins.

Cinnamon – is calming and helps to support healthy circulation and digestion.

Fennel – is very good for indigestion when served with honey

Ginseng – stimulates vitality and helps the body stay healthy.

Ginger root – is excellent for improving circulation, and is one of the best herbs for improving digestion, nausea, lung congestion, and arthritis.

Hawthorne – strengthens the heart and increases blood flow.

Hibiscus – helps sore throats, gum disease, cystitis and high blood pressure.

Juniper Berry – helps urinary problems and mixed with other berries is heart healthy

Lavender – promotes calmness. Best used in combination to avoid cramps.

Lemongrass – is frequently used due to its calming properties.

Lemon Myrtle – a fantastic cleanser for colds & flu.

Parsley – is a diuretic and helps with kidney function.

Pau d'arco - has anti-inflammatory and antimicrobial activity against a wide variety of organisms including bacteria, fungi, yeasts (including Candida albicans), viruses (including herpes simplex types I and II, influenza virus, poliovirus and retroviruses) and parasites.

Peppermint – is good for stress relief. It also helps with stomachs and digestive issues and helps to freshen the breath.

Red Clover - use as a medicine for menopausal symptoms, cancer, mastitis, joint disorders, asthma, bronchitis, psoriasis and eczema. It is not recommended for children, pregnant or breastfeeding women.

Raspberry Leaf – helps morning sickness and aids easier delivery.

Rose hips – are a natural source of vitamin C and bioflavonoid. They are a liver, kidney, and blood tonic, and are a good remedy for fatigue, colds, and cough.

Sage – fantastic for menopause and PMS.

Sarsaparilla – promotes energy and healthy skin.

Slippery elm – helps to relieve stomach cramps and other gastrointestinal problems.
Spearmint – good for upper respiratory conditions and sinuses.

Vervain - calm the nervous system and as a tonic for anxiety and mild depression.

Why use herbal teas?

No matter if you love herbal tea for its pleasurable taste, or if you just want the benefits it can provide for your health, herbal tea provides you with a plethora of choice! Here are some of the more common benefits they can provide.

- Achieving a more calm and relaxed state of mind

- Supporting heart health

- Aiding with stomach and digestive problems

- Providing cleansing properties for the body

- Promoting energy and wellness

- Nourishing the nervous system

- Strengthening the immune system

- Providing antioxidants to the body

- Boosting energy levels and invigorating the body

- Relieving stress
- Helping to avoid colds

- Stimulating the internal organs

- Promoting a good night's sleep

- And much more besides. Some of the more intricate ones are discussed below in more detail.

Relieves Joint Pain
Autoimmune joint dysfunction, which includes rheumatoid arthritis, is often a result of an over-reactive immune system and inflammation within our body. Several highly effective anti-inflammatory medicines are widely-used to deal with joint soreness; nevertheless they may well trigger a wide range of adverse effects. Examination conducted by the National Center of Complementary and Alternative Medicine implies that green tea herb possesses many anti-inflammatory characteristics that may help to greatly reduce the intensity of rheumatoid arthritis and other autoimmune ailments. Green tea is easily the most widely used herbal tea and is also referred to as Chinese tea or Japanese tea. While not typically a herbal tea, green tea is still beneficial. However note that it DOES contain caffeine.

Relieves Nausea
Natural herb teas such as ginger, lemon balm, red raspberry leaf and peppermint leaf teas are suggested by the American Pregnancy Association to decrease nausea, particularly while pregnant or maybe resulting from using medication. These kind of herbal teas help to control morning sickness and also other signs and symptoms of pregnancy, for example sleeplessness, fatigue, body swelling and irritable mood. Though these teas do not contain caffeine and are regarded beneficial for expecting mothers, it is very important talk to a health care provider before drinking herbal teas on a regular basis.

Helps Reduce Cholesterol and Weight
According to the Cleveland Clinic, numerous herbal teas could help lessen high cholesterol levels and even drop a few pounds. That is especially valuable for people that possess diabetes or heart disease or are obese. Herbal teas consisting of green tea, cinnamon, ephedra, garlic or hawthorn are believed to especially enhance circulation, lower dangerous levels of cholesterol and raise fat-burning in the abdomen

Treats Cold and Flu Symptoms
Herbal teas are likewise prominent for addressing cold and flu symptoms. Teas containing ginger, lemon, honey, ephedra, goldenseal, cinnamon, echinacea, peppermint or hyssops are typically

useful to minimize cold and flu symptoms for example inflamed throat, coughing, nasal congestion, sinus trouble and body aches. These herbal teas contain a lot of anti-inflammatory and antiviral attributes.

Promotes Healthy Sleep
Herbal teas are commonly put to use for supporting peaceful sleep and remedying sleep conditions much like insomnia. The National Center for Complementary and Alternative Medicine endorses chamomile, lime blossom, valerian and St. John's wort herbal teas for getting rid of the occasional insomnia issues. These teas consist of attributes which help relax the nerves, promote sleep and relieve muscle spasms.

And if all of that wasn't enough, your senses thank you when they are stimulated by herbal tea... the warmth of the cup in your hands... the visual pleasure in the vibrantly or delicately colored beverage... the aromatherapy of the delicious fragrance... and, finally, the calming deliciousness of the first taste!

Enough talk about what they are, let's find out how to make them...

How to make herbal tea

Making a great herbal tea is more or less an art you develop over time, how much water to use, how long to leave it steeping, how hot should the water be etc... All of these things, and many more, affect the overall quality texture and taste of your finished tea, but as with everything, there are several shortcuts of course.

When you are brewing your herbal tea, take advantage of fresh, cold water. Take care not to use aluminum cookware as it will have an impact on the quality. Take advantage of glass, cast iron, or stainless steel everywhere feasible. A tea strainer is tremendously effective since it lets you formulate your own personal blends of teas or herbs, and also blocks the leaves and flowers from escaping into the drink.

Boil one cup of water per person.

Now that the water has boiled, incorporate one heaped teaspoon of herbs for every single cup of water, either in individual cups, or in a teapot. Cover and let the herbs steep for five to ten minutes time. Be careful not to over-steep the herbs as the essence might become too strong and taste more medical-related rather than pleasurable, so for a new mixture test for taste every 3 minutes or so.

If you wish to enhance the flavor of your tea, honey or lemon can be fabulous possibilities.

To appropriately create herbal tea, use 1 tea bag per person or, in case you are making it from the dried herbs (and I hope that you are), use 1 teaspoon of the herb.

Herbal Tea Recipes

All Over Immunity

There are so many ways that our immune systems can be overwhelmed ... it's in our air, our water, our food, our workplace, our stress. This blend of organic and wild herbs is not only helpful but comforting, strengthening and tasty.

1 part red clover blossoms
1 part nettle leaves
1 part pau d'Arco
1 part alfalfa & sage leaves
1 part St.Johns wort tops
1 part ginger root

Place 1 teaspoon of herbs per cup in a tea ball or bag, put in your nicest or most favorite cup or mug, and cover with boiling water. Steep for 10 minutes. Remove tea ball or bag, and add sugar, honey, sweetener, milk, cream or whatever, to taste.

Allergy Shield

This tea maintains a cool minty, citrus flavor to assist you with the discomfort associated with allergy season.

1 part nettle
1 part peppermint
1 part spearmint
1 part yerba santa
1 part eyebright
1 pat lemongrass leaves
1 part calendula
1 part red clover
1 part lavender flowers
1 part fennel seeds
a pinch of stevia to sweeten

Place 1 teaspoon of herbs per cup in a tea ball or bag, put in your nicest or most favorite cup or mug, and cover with boiling water. Steep for 10 minutes. Remove tea ball or bag, and add sugar, honey, sweetener, milk, cream or whatever, to taste.

Aphrodite's Secret

A sensuous, aromatic blend with just the right tint of zest for your palate, and sure to kindle flames! A delicate, but dashing combination makes this one of your most enjoyable cups of tea. Can aid in boosting the libido of both sexes.

1 part Damiana leaves
1 part rose petals
1 part peppermint leaves
1 part muira puama
1 part gingko leaves
1 part orange peel
1 part cinnamon bark chips
pinch of stevia.

Place 1 teaspoon of herbs per cup in a tea ball or bag, put in your nicest or most favorite cup or mug, and cover with boiling water. Steep for 10 minutes. Remove tea ball or bag, and add sugar, honey, sweetener, milk, cream or whatever, to taste.

Blood Booster

When you have a low iron count then you can feel rough, this tea stops that.

1 tsp Rose Hips-crushed
1 Tsp Butcher's Broom
1 Tsp Yellow Dock

Bring 3 1/2 cups of water to a boil. Remove water from heat and add herbs. Place a tight lid on the pot. Let the mixture steep for five to ten minutes. Drink one cup three times daily. Yields three cups.

Blooming Healthy

Beautiful to look at, nectar to taste and good for you. A popular tea. Spirited, uplifting and energizing.

1 part ginkgo leaves
1 part red clover tops
1 part nettle leaves
1 part meadowsweet leaves
1 part calendula
2 parts chamomile
2 parts lavender flowers
1 part gotu kola leaves
a pinch of stevia.

Place 1 teaspoon of herbs per cup in a tea ball or bag, put in your nicest or most favorite cup or mug, and cover with boiling water. Steep for 10 minutes. Remove tea ball or bag, and add sugar, honey, sweetener, milk, cream or whatever, to taste.

Blues Tea

Fights depression and monthly mental fatigue.

1 part Nettle leaves,
1 part St Johns wort tops
2 parts spearmint
1 part damiana leaves
1 part kava kava root
a tiny pinch of stevia to taste

Place 1 teaspoon of herbs per cup in a tea ball or bag, put in your nicest or most favorite cup or mug, and cover with boiling water. Steep for 10 minutes. Remove tea ball or bag, and add sugar, honey, sweetener, milk, cream or whatever, to taste.

Calm Waters

Just a simple and easy tea to help calm the mind and body.

2 parts Lemon balm
2 parts Chamomile flowers
1 part St Johns Wort

Place 2 tablespoons of herbs for each cup, in a tea ball or bag, put in your nicest or most favorite cup or mug, and cover with boiling water. Steep for 10 minutes. Remove tea ball or bag, and add sugar, honey, sweetener, milk, cream or whatever, to taste.

Colds and Flu Tea

The name says it all.

1 part Blackberry leaves
1 part Elder flowers
1 part Linden flowers
1 part Peppermint leaves

Place 2 tablespoons of herbs for each cup, in a tea ball or bag, put in your nicest or most favorite cup or mug, and cover with boiling water. Steep for 10 minutes. Remove tea ball or bag, and add sugar, honey, sweetener, milk, cream or whatever, to taste.

Dry, raspy cough

Nobody likes having an irritating cough, so blend this tea together and sip it throughout the day when needed.

1 part Licorice Root
1 part Slippery Elm
1 part Mullein
1 part Catnip
1 part Chamomile
Honey
Lemon 1 wedge

Place 2 tablespoons of herbs for each cup, in a tea ball or bag, put in your nicest or most favorite cup or mug, and cover with boiling water. Steep for 10 minutes. Remove tea ball or bag, and add sugar, honey, sweetener, milk, cream or whatever, to taste.

Detoxification Tea

Not typically a herbal tea in its strictest sense, however when brewed and sipped throughout the day it does a great job of detoxing the body.

1 part Green Tea leaves

Place 1 teaspoon of herbs per cup in a tea ball or bag, put in your nicest or most favorite cup or mug, and cover with boiling water. Steep for 10 minutes. Remove tea ball or bag, and add sugar, honey, sweetener, milk, cream or whatever, to taste.

Epilepsy Combination

Never a replacement for correct medication, however in severe cases it can be helpful to relax and tame seizures and in some cases even prevents them. Sip as needed throughout the day.

1 part Valerian
1 part Skullcap
1 part Hops

Place 1 teaspoon of herbs per cup in a tea ball or bag, put in your nicest or most favorite cup or mug, and cover with boiling water. Steep for 10 minutes. Remove tea ball or bag, and add sugar, honey, sweetener, milk, cream or whatever, to taste.

Fever Reducer Tea

When a fever strikes then you know that the body is already well under attack. Drinking this tea will help to stave off the infection and bring the body back to normal, fast.

2 parts dried Catnip
1 part dry Vervain

Place 1 teaspoon of herbs per cup in a tea ball or bag, put in your nicest or most favorite cup or mug, and cover with boiling water. Steep for 10 minutes. Remove tea ball or bag, and add sugar, honey, sweetener, milk, cream or whatever, to taste.

Fluid Retention Tea

Every woman knows the benefits of losing excess fluids in the body, to reveal a lighter, healthier and happier you.

3 parts Dandelion root
3 parts Dandelion leaves
2 parts Nettle leaves
2 parts Spearmint leaves

Place 1 teaspoon of herbs per cup in a tea ball or bag, put in your nicest or most favorite cup or mug, and cover with boiling water. Steep for 10 minutes. Remove tea ball or bag, and add sugar, honey, sweetener, milk, cream or whatever, to taste.

Happy Man Tea Blend

Any man knows how important to keep their 'equipment' in top notch order so it works as expected. This tea helps to repair damage and keep everything working correctly.

1 part Siberian ginseng
1 part dandelion root
1 part nettle
1 part each marshmallow & burdock roots
1 part each hawthorn & saw palmetto berries
1 part fennel seeds
1 part wildoats
a pinch of stevia

Place 1 teaspoon of herbs per cup in a tea ball or bag, put in your nicest or most favorite cup or mug, and cover with boiling water. Steep for 10 minutes. Remove tea ball or bag, and add sugar, honey, sweetener, milk, cream or whatever, to taste. Climb into bed and enjoy!

Happy Tummy Tea

Put a smile on your face with this soothing and yummy tea.

1 part catnip
1 part spearmint & lemongrass leaves
1 part calendula flowers
1 part skullcap
1 part rosemary & sage leaves
1 part fennel seeds

Place 1 teaspoon of herbs per cup in a tea ball or bag, put in your nicest or most favorite cup or mug, and cover with boiling water. Steep for 10 minutes. Remove tea ball or bag, and add sugar, honey, sweetener, milk, cream or whatever, to taste.

Heartburn Tea

Prepare and drink when you have heartburn.

1 tablespoon Chamomile
1 table spoon Peppermint
2 pods Star Anise

Boil pods for 5 minutes. Place 1 teaspoon of herbs per cup in a tea ball or bag, put in your nicest or most favorite cup or mug, and cover with boiling water. Steep for 10 minutes. Remove tea ball or bag, and add sugar, honey, sweetener, milk, cream or whatever, to taste.

Less Stress Tea

Relieves stress, relaxes low back and neck areas.

1 part chamomile
1 part mint
1 part calendula flowers

Place 1 teaspoon of herbs per cup in a tea ball or bag, put in your nicest or most favorite cup or mug, and cover with boiling water. Steep for 10 minutes. Remove tea ball or bag, and add sugar, honey, sweetener, milk, cream or whatever, to taste.

Memory Zest Blend

A mentally refreshing beverage, to help give you feelings of clarity

and precision.
1 part ginkgo
1 part gotu kola and peppermint leaves
1 part red clover tops
1 part rosemary leaves
1 part ginger root
a pinch of stevia.

Place 1 teaspoon of herbs per cup in a tea ball or bag, put in your nicest or most favorite cup or mug, and cover with boiling water. Steep for 10 minutes. Remove tea ball or bag, and add sugar, honey, sweetener, milk, cream or whatever, to taste.

Nausea Tea

Thankfully we don't often get nauseous, but when we do, it's nice to know we can do something about it.

1 part dried Ginger root
1 part Clove blossoms
2 parts Chamomile flowers

Place 1 teaspoon of herbs per cup in a tea ball or bag, put in your nicest or most favorite cup or mug, and cover with boiling water. Steep for 10 minutes. Remove tea ball or bag, and add sugar, honey, sweetener, milk, cream or whatever, to taste.

Nervous Stomach Tea

Sometimes in life we reach a point where our anxiety overwhelms our physiological functions, usually resulting in a nervous stomach. Drink when required until symptoms stop.

4 parts Angelica root
4 parts Lemon Balm leaves
1 part Fennel seed

Bring Angelica root to a simmer in 4 cups water. Turn off heat, add lemon balm & lemon; steep 10 minutes & strain.

Quiet Time Tea

When you just need to relax a bit and forget what's going on in the world.

1 part oregano
2 parts Chamomile
1 part lemon balm
1 part lemon thyme

Place 1 teaspoon of herbs per cup in a tea ball or bag, put in your nicest or most favorite cup or mug, and cover with boiling water. Steep for 10 minutes. Remove tea ball or bag, and add sugar, honey, sweetener, milk, cream or whatever, to taste.

Sleep Tea Recipe

Insomnia causes so many problems that it's hard to start to count them all, but it doesn't have to be that way.

2 parts Hops
1 part Lavender
1 part Rosemary
1 part Thyme
1 part Mugwort
1 part Sage
1 Pinch of Valerian Root

Place 1 teaspoon of herbs per cup in a tea ball or bag, put in your nicest or most favorite cup or mug, and cover with boiling water. Steep for 10 minutes. Remove tea ball or bag, and add sugar, honey, sweetener, milk, cream or whatever, to taste.

Sore throat

Known to soothe a sore throat when sipped throughout the day.

1 part Licorice root
1 part Slippery Elm
1 part Peppermint

Place 1 teaspoon of herbs per cup in a tea ball or bag, put in your nicest or most favorite cup or mug, and cover with boiling water. Steep for 10 minutes. Remove tea ball or bag, and add sugar, honey, sweetener, milk, cream or whatever, to taste.

Super Relaxer Tea

This is great at night before bed

1 part (1 teaspoon) valerian root (dried)
1 part (1 teaspoon)Chamomile flowers (dried)

Place 1 teaspoon of herbs per cup in a tea ball or bag, put in your nicest or most favorite cup or mug, and cover with boiling water. Steep for 10 minutes. Remove tea ball or bag, and add sugar, honey, sweetener, milk, cream or whatever, to taste.

Tea for Health

A general tonic to keep you healthy.

1 part China black tea
2 part fennel
1 part mint
2 parts rose hips
1 part elder flower
2 parts hops
1 part mullein

Place 1 teaspoon of herbs per cup in a tea ball or bag, put in your nicest or most favorite cup or mug, and cover with boiling water. Steep for 10 minutes. Remove tea ball or bag, and add sugar, honey, sweetener, milk, cream or whatever, to taste.

Tea for menstrual problems, fertility and childbirth.

3 tablespoons sassafras bark
2 tablespoons dandelion root
1 tablespoon ginger root
½ tablespoon cinnamon
1 tablespoon licorice root
½ tablespoon orange peel
1 tablespoon pau d'arco
¼ tablespoon dong quai root
1 tablespoon chaste berry
1 tablespoon wild yam

Place 1 teaspoon of herbs per cup in a tea ball or bag, put in your nicest or most favorite cup or mug, and cover with boiling water. Steep for 10 minutes. Remove tea ball or bag, and add sugar, honey, sweetener, milk, cream or whatever, to taste.

Upset Stomach Tea

For when you need to function normally but your body won't let you.

1 part Peppermint leaves
1 part Lemon Balm leaves
1 part Fennel seeds

Place 1 teaspoon of herbs per cup in a tea ball or bag, put in your nicest or most favorite cup or mug, and cover with boiling water. Steep for 10 minutes. Remove tea ball or bag, and add sugar, honey, sweetener, milk, cream or whatever, to taste.

Winter Tea

Helps fend off the changes in weather, central heating damage, bugs, viruses and general nasty stuff.

1 part Boneset
1 part Echinacea
1 part Peppermint

Place 1 teaspoon of herbs per cup in a tea ball or bag, put in your nicest or most favorite cup or mug, and cover with boiling water. Steep for 10 minutes. Remove tea ball or bag, and add sugar, honey, sweetener, milk, cream or whatever, to taste.

Very Odd Cure for Bad Breath

Drink tea.

Researchers from the College of Dentistry at the University of Illinois at Chicago say compounds in tea can slow the growth of bacteria in our mouths, which is the primary cause of bad breath. The magic ingredients are antioxidants called polyphenols, and they are found in both green and black teas.

It's the bacteria that live on the back surface of the tongue and in the deep pockets between the gums and teeth that make our breath smell bad. The bacteria "make horrible, smelly stuff," lead study author Christine D. Wu explained to Reuters in an interview. "That's why we get bad breath." Wu and her colleagues showed in earlier studies that black tea can slow dental plaque formation and help your toothpaste work more effectively.

Her latest laboratory experiments have shown that tea's polyphenols not only inhibit three species of bacteria that cause halitosis, but also stop an enzyme that causes the formation of hydrogen sulfide--the ultimate culprit for rotten breath.

But here's the catch: Tea won't sweeten your breath. So don't throw out the mouthwash just yet. "All we can say is that a cup of tea will produce more than enough of these active materials to affect the bacteria," she said. "Remember, this is a lab study. In the mouth, bacteria are protected by all sorts of things."

Bonus herbal smoothie recipes

Berry Basil Green

Cool, crisp and outrageously tasty.

The Ingredients
1 cup water
1 fresh or frozen banana
1 cup spinach
6-8 fresh basil leaves
1 cup fresh or frozen berries (blackberries, blueberries, raspberries, strawberries, or a combo)
1 tablespoon coconut oil
A dash of cinnamon
A little honey, maple syrup, or stevia to sweeten

Put all ingredients into a blender and blitz until smooth. Serve immediately.

Raspberry Rosemary

A traditional taste which you won't forget.

The Ingredients
1 cup water
1 cup frozen raspberries
1/2 cup frozen blueberries or blackberries
1-2 sprigs fresh rosemary, leaves removed and finely chopped
A little honey to sweeten (optional)
1/2 fresh or frozen banana

Put all ingredients into a blender and blitz until smooth. Serve immediately.

Strawberry Mint Green

Very, very appetizing, with a kick

The Ingredients
1 and 1/2 cups water
1 fresh or frozen banana
1 cup fresh or frozen strawberries
1 cup spinach, kale, or other leafy green
1-2 tablespoons dried and powdered down mint leaves, or 6-8 fresh mint leaves
A little honey, maple syrup, or stevia to sweeten (optional)

Put all ingredients into a blender and blitz until smooth. Serve immediately.

Hot and Spicy Green

When you want something a bit more fiery.

The Ingredients
1 and 1/2 cups of water
1/2 avocado
1-2 cups kale or spinach
1/2 cup fresh or frozen blueberries
1 tablespoon chia seeds or chia seed gel
1 tablespoon coconut oil
1/4 teaspoon chili powder
A little honey, maple syrup, or stevia to sweeten (optional)
1/3 cup coconut flakes or shreds

Put all ingredients into a blender and blitz until smooth. Serve immediately.

Get Your 100% Free Recipes & Formulations

Don't forget, to get your free recipes and much, much more, simply head on over to

http://ross.theherbalworkshop.co.uk

Send us your email and first name and I will ensure that you get fantastic value for money with ongoing, free recipes and formulations in our spectacular herbal health newsletter.

Jessica Ross

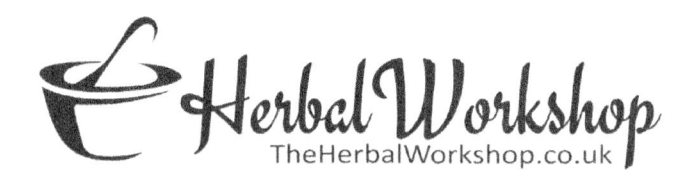

Other books of interest

How to Make Tinctures and heal your body naturally

Written by: Jessica Ross
Amazon ASIN: B00FMYO07S

Drift into the fantastically aromatic field of remedial tinctures and expose an alternative, balanced you. Uplift your spirits, restore your present health, and take pleasure in absolute tranquility. Written for the beginner and advanced user alike.

How to Grow Strawberries Using Only Organic Methods

Written by: Laura Crouch
Amazon ASIN: B00FRH48DQ

Before you start thinking that growing strawberries must be too hard otherwise everybody will be doing it, it's easier than you could imagine. Dirt, plants and a bit of care is all you need to grow a bounty of delicious and nutritious dessert that your neighborhood will be envious of and your neighbors will desire.

How to Cook Strawberry – 20 foolproof, easy, fast & cheap recipes

Written by: Antoine Rochelle
Amazon ASIN: B00FRHA44I

Strawberries. The small, squishy red fruit that has been coveted by generations. Why does the tantalizing, sweet little berry tempt us so much? Why do we see it as a sign of summer and of lavish desserts? Whatever the reason, making desserts with them transforms them from decadent fruits into total temptation for your taste buds.

Printed in Great Britain
by Amazon